The Miracle of Anti ageing

    As a man you will walk in a good stride, to the envy of your peers.
    As a woman you will radiate a nebula of youth and beauty, to be question?

Emilio Garcia

Copy right 2009 by Emilio Garcia
All rights reserved

THERE IS NO CURE FOR DISEASE, ONLY REMISSION, AND PREVENTION.

    Aging is an aberration of the human herd phenomenon, through pathologic disease.
    The human being, is a carnivore, you are an animal. your descendants go back one hundred and sixty five million years.

HUMAN PARASITES OF PLANET EARTH.

You are the macro parasite of planet earth. In your existence, you have driven into extinction, count less numbers of life forms. humans are capable of killing off its own species. humans move in groups, interacting with other groups, of its own species, trading goods, maintaining border guards, protecting its bounders, attacking its neighbors, pure natural animal instincts. Its leadership phoneme is natural in the entire animal world. Its consuming alcohol and other drugs, throughout history accounts for its abnormal behavior.

The drugs, and chemicals, it consumes today, has evolved. Its effects are new abnormal behaviors, and diseases. The fact of the matter is that you are part of an animal herd, roaming the earth. Just because you are reading this book, means nothing. It cannot change what you are. what you are doing on this planet. or the effect you have on this planet. It is because you are a parasite, you have manage to come this far. your technology is from the after math, of world wars, and millions of humans killed. the jet plane, rocket, the atomic bomb, industrial farming, the killing off, the sacrifices of wild plant and animal life, for a few good crops, and domesticated animals.

Understanding what you are, why you are on this planet, and how you affect this planet. Will give you some incites into why you are ageing. you are a human herd animal, and all animal herds, must maintain the strong, and the weak, old, and infirm, die off.

Humans under the skin are a sophisticated unimaginable bio chemical electrical invormental adapting interacting systems; bent on survival. spanning a million year struggle. humans would not survive a second, if they could not utilize, convert, and neutralize, chemicals, food, and larger macro parasites, on this planet.

In this struggle, there is no place for the weak, old and infirm. In this struggle, the unimaginable bio chemical electrical adapting interacting human system. through the success of the human species. understands this well. as your usefulness, as a young strong person, moves in time. a system that is the prorogation of the species. through its gene processes.

At thirty-five years of age, genes in the body, begin to turn off all the essential amino acids. that stimulates, the growth hormones, arginine, tyrosine, glyine etc; at fifty-five years of age, the human growth hormone that accounts for strong muscle energy, and repairing damage tissue. does not exist, in the body. genes turn off the pituitary glands, growth hormone production processes. causing a decline in the thymus gland. throughout the body, enzymes, nutrients, amino acids, hormones. that support life, and prevent body damage, are turned off. this condition is trigger by the slow bio feed back, of a biological awareness. the graying hair, tried feeling, the lack of collagen support, the spiraling consciences of getting old and impending death. this cannot, in the final analyses be prevented, with today's science.

TRADITIONAL MEDICINE

The whole is the sum of its parts. is the illusion that dominates traditional medicine? and entire western consciences. humans are far from machines. you and I shall take a journey into the real world of human health, and prevention. a dirty word, because there is no money to be made in health prevention. there are billions of dollars that are being made in treating symptoms, and selling prescription drugs. in a corrupt food, and pharmaceutical regulated industries. that disrupts the chemical and interacting balance of human chemistry. the egotistic assumption, that one can understand the biological complexities of human chemistry. by isolation, and not understand, the more important chemical, neurochemistry, electrical interactions, is absurd. the effect of this tunnel vision mentally. is a mad painful rush, to certain death.

How are you friend, fellow carnivore, you are not shocked, buy all of this, you know it, you feel it, you understand it, you just do not talk about it, do you.

Let us take one-step back; you think you are a special entity. you even have a spiritual mental frame of reference, you cannot believe you are just a herd animal. you are Gods flock are you not?

THE HUMAN HERD ANIMAL

The human being is after all a herd animal, and herds, gather in groups, as part of a group, the individuals mentality regress to a primitive, and a leader will emerge, in a complex society, individuals that share a discontent, will band together in groups for many causes. the leader of all groups will lead the group to kill, or help, as in the KKK or NAACP etc. the difference in human herd animals, and other herd animals are that the human understands, it has a past, and a human contemplates its future. other herd animals live in the present,
they do not worry they are ruminators.

And you though you were going to find a little magic pill, or a food list, that would make you young. my dear friend you live in the chemical invasion epoch.

THE CHEMICAL INVASION EPOCH

Mankind's genetic structure has changed little, in one hundred thousand years. and can only survive with a diet genetically correct.

For the last twenty thousand years. humans have consumed mostly real fruits, and vegetables, and occasionally meat. In the last fifty years, humans consume millions of tons of harmful chemicals, called food, drugs, and air.

Humans are and amazing adaptable species. are dieing off by the millions, in today's chemical invasion epoch.

Humans are not poised, to sudden change. and will not survive another thousand years. due to the chemical invasion epoch, and the genetically evolve viruses in immunosuppressed patients. this book is about anti ageing, not the imbecility of human politics. the drug effected rich people, with identity problems. that make inept decisions.

This book is about the few lucky people like you that are reading this book; there are more then one hundred million people in pain today; in western society. a hundred million people will not read this book. most of them will suffer the demise of harmful chemicals, in food, drugs, and air. that causes arthritis, diabetes, cancer, gallstones, hemorrhoids, high cholesterol, high blood pressure, rheumatoid arthritis, infertility, lupus, and heart attacks.

Their doctor will give them one form of opiate, that they can leave this world. a drug addict, stoned out of their mines.

You my dear friend may not share that fate. if you are willing to give up the food, you love to eat, and eat real food. to supplement and rebuild the body, as it degenerates, from the genetic process of killing off the old. if you have a will to live, the strength to break away from the herd, its mores, that perpetuate early painful or sudden death. then I shall give on to you, and awakening.

THE AWAKENING

The sun is breaking though night, it is early morning, carbon monoxide fills the air, the sound of cars, and trucks, can be heard, they are starting to back up streets and highways. two hundred million human herd animals, move on to trains buses streets and highways. they walk amongst the sick, virus infected, diseased, and dieing fellow workers. they gather by the millions, at dirty, filthy, coffee shops and restaurants. the caffeine junkies have coffee and a donut or bagel, maybe an egg sandwich, juice, a cigarette.

Caffeine is a powerful addictive drug, a slightly bitter alkaloid. 1.3.7 trimethylxanthine. It stimulates the sympathetic nervous system. fooling the brain, by filling receptors in place of adenosine, making a person think he or she is alert. caffeine addicts in time suffer from sleep deprivation. humans need to sleep. It is one important aspect of good health and long life. sleep deprivation will weaken the immune system. leaving you susceptible to disease.

The tap water that is used to make coffee. at the dirty coffee shop, has chemicals collectively called trihalomethanes, thirty-two known to cause cancer, heavy metals, runoffs from highways that are salted, sanded, or nitrates from fertilizes lands.

The donut and bagel was made with cheap white flour

with cancer causing chemicals, like BHT. at lunch, millions of human herd animals gather in groups at dirty luncheonettes. they wolf down so-called food sandwiches loaded with salt that gives them high blood pressure.

    The vegetables and disserts have cancer causing preservatives, additives and food colors. the meat and cold cuts have diethylstilbestrol, and sodium nitrate, known to cause cancer. the caffeine is a stimulant; the refined sugar gives you hyperglycemia. you feel tired, and excited, you do not want to go back to work. you want to go to sleep. at work, you have another cup of coffee, three sugars, you feel a bit of heartburn, and you take an antacid.

    Antacids can cause hypochlorhydria. (overgrowth of helicobacter pylori) many diseases are associated with impaired gastric acid. dirty luncheonettes, are associated with diseases like cancer. you are the working animal, in the phoneme of sociological human herd animal behavior. you leave work and again, are amongst the sick, virus infected, diseased and dieing fellow workers.   at home, you have dinner, a steak, vegetables, coffee, sports T V, beer, wake up tired and beat.

    Their must be a better way to make a living. your protruding belly, you attribute to good health. your mental frame of reference is nothing less then deplorable, liberalism. that allows you to rationalize the fact that you gulp down chemical garbage you call food. and spit out true Hegelian rhetoric, life is what it is accepting your fate. when it is your time to go, you go. everything that is going on is right,

DELUSIONAL LIBERALS

My defiant, delusional, liberal friend. you are a barrel shaped person sitting on a train, racing, to an unavoidable train wreak. there you will experience disease, pain, and sudden death.

For those of you that are not so liberal mined. the time has come to talk of many things of life of death. of those that exploit the weak liberal mine, for greed and profit. I must apologize for coming down so hard on you base liberals. when it is surely the opposite. the men and women that are infected with Nietzsche's calling, a will to power. that process cheap chemicals call it food, hire a role model that would eat the so-called food, in a TV commercial. and feed it to all accepting open mouthed, liberals. for love of power and money. are indeed the bad people, but are they the bad people, you have a choice. you live in a great democracy, no one can force you to eat or not eat garbage.

You do it because you love the way it taste. you condemn no one; your lax mental state is conditioned by your religion. thou shall not, and the true sprit of Hegel's philosophy.

AGEING

Ageing is an aberration of the human herd phenomena through pathologic disease. if you are a creature of western society, you probably have a disease or a health condition. you must be free of disease, or any adverse health condition. this book will address disease. will give you an awareness of your disease. that you may work with your health care professional, as a team of two specialists. you must understand your therapy, side effects, of all drugs, and make the final decision, in what therapy or drugs to take, or not to take. and not under the threat of death. that is the critique of most health care professionals. to convince you to take drugs, therapy, or surgery. that in most cases promotes the spiraling degeneration, of ill health and painful death.

One cannot think in terms of anti aging and be affected by disease. I am free of disease, or any adverse health condition. I look twenty years younger then I am. I welcome you to take this journey with me. to have an optimistic mental frame of reference. knowing you can overcome prevent and hold the precious gift of good health and long life.

As people reach middle age in western society. are affected by one or another form of systemic, autoimmune, rheumatic diseases. arthritis etc. the contradiction of this statement is juvenile rheumatic arthritis, systemic lupus erythematosus, juvenile spondyloarthropathies, and juvenile dermatomyositis all caused by the chemcial invasion epoch, we live in. and the human genes that turn off, the life sustaining hormones, enzymes, and nutrients, as time goes by. again, there are no magic pills.

    Are you so inept to think that you are not an animal, you communicate with other animals of your species. through language an interaction of speech, smell, site, and body language. you breathe in air, to process oxygen. your body reacts to everything that is in the air, that you breathe. you cannot deny, that you are a bio chemical electrical invormental interacting species. and what affects this animal will determine your health, and how long you will be with us, on this planet.

    With this understanding, all disease can go into remission. In addition, one can begin the journey. if you believe your disease and state of health is self-perpetrating. read no more, give this book to a higher intellect.

    Seek out the practitioners of spare parts, and gadgets, the thinkers of reductionism, in traditional medicine, and may GOD save you from eminent pain and sudden death, for I have spoken.

UNDERSTANDING THE CAUSE OF AGEING

The issue is before you, for the few that are left with me. we now have a clear understanding of the cause of ageing, disease, and premature death. we move on to repairing damage human cells, regenerating cells, reinforcing cells, maintaining the health of all cells, neutralizing harmful chemicals, replacing lost nutrients, and amino acids, stimulating the body, to produce natural hormones that the body turns off. in the process of eliminating the weak, that the strong will perpetuate the species. remission of all adverse conditions. strengthen all major organs, and restoring, supporting, maintaining, enhancing, the most importing system of the body, the immune system. that will take you out of pain.

you live in the chemical invasion epoch. the cause of disease. you understand it, you will eat none of it.

THE OPTIMIST

You need to have an optimistic mental frame of reverence. you have just won the lottery of good health. "congratulations" because you are an interacting creature. positive, psycho semantic and bio feed back, can improve your health. It is a scientific fact that your state of mine will have and effect on your health.

THE IMMUNE SYSTEM

I must say in a hundred and sixty five million years from human conception. the human immune system would not, could not, and did not. attack a healthy cell.

The immune system has evolved over millions of years to protect the body. then why would it destroy cells and tissue, it attacks cells and tissue, because something is affecting the cell, or tissue. and the integrity of the cell or tissue is challenge. the immune system treats it as defected cell, and destroys it. cancer cells, virus infected cells, bacteria infected tissue, infected cells, cells that are infected by free radicals, harmful chemicals and alleges.

We must assists the immune system, by neutralizing, and eliminate what is adversely affecting cells. this done, the immune system will not attack tissue or cells. and you are out of pain, and in remission.

Doctors address this problem in reverse, they try to suppress the pain, with harmful drugs, then they try to suppress the immune system, with harmful drugs, I am not going to list the harmful drugs doctors use. I am sure you are aware of them, if not taking them as I speak. this traditional approach to rheumatic diseases is appalling. if your house was invaded, in the process of being robbed, and destroyed, would you turn off the alarm. and if the police were on their way to try to prevent this. would you try to stop them, from entering your house? if you accomplish this, your house would surely be destroyed.

You know, you are not getting better. your condition is not improving, you need more drugs, to suppress the pain. in addition, the drugs that suppress your immune system. are making you sick, you are depressed, and you are praying for help. my dear friend it is not such a big problem. obviously, your immune system is overworking, trying to naturalize bad chemicals, carcinogens, destroying tissues, and cells that are affected by all this. stop, pay attention, your life is on the line. you look terrible, over weight, tired, in pain; you are worried you may suffer a heart attack. and need bypass surgery. the food industry calling everything they sell natural. no one knows if the food is real food, it is natural chemicals, natural color, and natural sugar. (do I still have your attention)

STRESS

most people that live in western society share the same stress. in personal health, and world politics, our health care system, and its practitioners are as illusional as the drugs they use. that do not work.

If every one had government paid, free health care, it would create   cataclysmic events that would, beckon the fall of an already bankrupt national economy. due to the fact that millions of new cases of heart disease, cancer, diabetes, and all the related diseases, of the chemical invasion epoch, we live in today.

WAR STRATEGY

Our political leaders' have no idea of grand strategy; one cannot confront an enemy, a terrorist of gorilla warfare, or a dictator. that would be considered a frontal attack, like storming a castile. you cannot win. you win the war by cutting supply lines. and attacking the enemy in the rear. all wars, in all of human history, were won, in the implementation and understanding of this grand strategy. take the Korean dictator, he test a nuclear bomb, our leaders confront him, with political rhetoric and concern. when what should be done, is demand that china, stop supplying Korea, so that the government of Korea shall fall, and not be a treat to world peace. alternatively, we must break all ties, with china, stop all trade, with china, and consider china a treat to world peace. understanding our grand strategy, we force china to cut all supply lines to Korea the war is won.

Our political leaders are drug addicts. the surgeon general of the United States issued the warning that nicotine is as addictive as heroin or cocaine. smoking is extremely toxic. toxic chemicals accumulate in the brain. alters brain chemicals. and severely disrupt normal function. smokers with every puff breathe in poisonous carbon monoxide

Let us move on to more important things, for none of this will matter if you are dead. the immune system is important, and every day stress can have an adverse affect. be it mental or fiscal, of cause what can be done about the ill-informed leaders of our great government. (the rich people with identity problems,) that make inept decisions. not much, let us hope they go away in time, and are replaced with more informed rich people. with identity problems. before we lose the war,

    As for stress it is quite simple. neutralizes stress, every day take. 1,500 mg of valerian root extract, two times a day. and before you go to bed, take 200mg of kava. If you are old, add 3mg of melatonin a half hour before bedtime. you will be relaxed and sleep like a rock. and the stress of every day life will be gone, the imbecility of human politics will still be their, but it will not affect your immune system. therefore, my friend in the process of anti aging, we must first put and end to stress.

    The scourge of mankind, the perpetuation of anger, heart disease, guilt feeling, fatigue, constipation, headaches, nervousness, asthma, ulcers, sleep deprivation, (no thanks, I stop drinking coffee.) to much caffeine burns up vitamin B in your body, everyone needs vitamin B to calm the nerves, aid digestion, good heart function, good vision, hair, and skin. calms the aching muscles, regenerate blood cells, and foremost maintains a healthy liver. no coffee for me; a bottle of spring water thank you.

    How can I walk along the seashore? take deep breaths, sit relaxed, and meditate, listen to the relaxing music of the ocean, drinking a cup of Siberian ginseng tea, for the sole purpose ending stress in my body. when you put dangerous drugs, like caffeine in soda, chocolate, and so many products. if I were not intelligent enough, to be aware of the chemical invasion epoch, I live in. I would be a nervous wreck, suffering from a bad case of insomnia. suffer memory loss, depression, problems in my relationships, from and over dose of caffeine, and a related vitamin B deficiency.

BY PASS SURGERY

Did you really need that by pass surgery? there is a lot of evidence, that our health care system is performing unnecessary surgery. you have a pain, you go to your doctor, and he says you have a build up in your artery. If we do not operate right away, you may die. why anyone would put you under the knife. in such a dangerous procedure, that would leave you cripple, or even dead. then put you on anticoagulants, that cause more problems then you started with. (one hundred thousand dollars) millions of Americans have heart disease. and a million new cases every year. all can be reversed, and in remission with out surgery.

Let me give you a treat. I will take a pound of over refined cheap flour that has no nutritional value. a lot of refined sugar that will make you fat. orange food color that will give you asthma, an allergies. add some chemicals BHT, BHA, that may cause cancer. cook all this good stuff, in cheap coconut or vegetable oil, trans fatty acids, only 0.5grams of TFAs if the label says in really small print only 0.5grams of TFAs don't buy it, it will kill you in time. but then, maybe, you will eat it, because it is all natural. and has no cholesterol (the evil word) it is ok to eat anything that has no cholesterol. the chemicals, the garbage food, just shovel it down your mouth.

Do not worry, it has no cholesterol. I could put a label, no cholesterol on road kill. and someone would put in on the barbeque. with the other dead animals.

Before your doctor cuts you in half. in the bacteria resistant, staph infection, operating room. did he not tell you that, the cholesterol build up in your artery? is their to protect your artery. (the injury hypothesis) you think if you eat cholesterol, that's the problem, eating cholesterol has nothing to do with it. the body produces cholesterol that sticks to the walls of your arteries. as part of a patch, over an injury, other parts may be muscle cells, connective tissue, platelets, called plaque, and if the patch gets big enough. it will stop the blood flow, what is the injury, your thinking. it is from the chemicals in what your smoking, drinking, eating, breathing, free radicals, trans fats, in your diet, and the chemicals your body produces under stress. what doctors call endothelial vessel layer injury? or atherosclerotic lesions. I kid you not, my friend, as much as you try to lower your (evil word) cholesterol. the body produces enough cholesterol to keep you healthy. and help to repair damaged arteries.

So lowering your cholesterol has nothing to do with blocked arteries, your doctor did not tell you; it's a sick society we live in, can't trust anyone any more, not even your own doctor.

You cannot grow old, if they cut you in half, and reroute a few arteries. this will not stop the cause of future damage. how many times can they cut you in half? and reroute arteries,

for love of money. your doctor tells you, you have heart disease, and if you do not have bypass surgery, you will die. take the alternative IV chelation therapy. It removes the calcium, in the plaque, that is clogging your arteries. and works as an anticoagulant. IV chelation therapy will address the problem. and will save you, eighty thousand dollars, and your life. fifty percent of bypass patients die in, or not long after surgery. Chelation therapy, used in as late as 1950 as a treatment for lead poisoning. (EDTA) is put into the body, in an I V, in a vein, bines with all the bad metals. And is carried out of the body through the urine.

Bypass, the bypass surgery. and address the cause and prevent the damage. there is no profit in prevention you have to spend money. think of the one hundred thousand dollars you will save, and the pain you will not suffer.

to reduce arterial plaque, expand blood vessels, and inhibit the blood clotting factor. I V chelation therapy is a good alternative to bypass surgery. doctors have known about this for many years. then why is it not recommended. I V chelation therapy cost a few thousand dollars. a bypass can cost ninety thousand dollars, and more after surgery, if you are still around, you do the math.

To maintain healthy blood vessels, you need to increase the nitric oxide levels, in the blood.   take a complex of the amino acids. (L-arginine and L-citrulline) safe at recommended doses. you can buy it on line.

To maintain healthy blood vessels. the essential amino acid, (L-Lysine) 500mg per day. works to utilize fatty acids, and conserve calcium. and added benefit prevents herpes simplex virus from replicating (cold sores). safe at recommend doses.

For vital oxygen take (L- carnitine) in other countries, it is prescribed for congestive heart failure. helps get vital oxygen to the heart. people with heart problems take high doses, like 3 grams with no side effects. I take 500mg per day,

THE SURVIVAL GENETIC FACTOR

to prevent heart problems. the body produces amino acids less, as time goes by, due to what I call the survival genetic factor. that is the genes turning off vital amino acids. killing off the old.

genes turning off the life support systems. that the young may perpetuate the species.

IF NOT PREVENT AGEING   SLOW ITS   PROCESS.
move fats out of cells. and maintain the integrity of cells. an works as a neurotransmitter. take (Lecithin with phosphatidyl choline) no side effects.

It is important to understand the free radical theory of aging. and to naturalizes the damage to the walls of artery's. from lipid per oxidation, caused by harmful chemicals. the pressing need to supplement, with natural vitamin E 800mg selenium 200mg and vitamin C 1,000mg. taken together, to synthesize, and producing a powerful antioxidant. is in it self the essence of long life. In today's chemical invasion epoch.

In the final analysis, the heart is an inconceivable bio chemical, electoral, pumping apparatus. however, for your Newtonian mentally, just a pump.

CELL ENERGY

A pump that needs a lot of energy. the body produces a nutrient, an energy component of every cell in the body. as time goes by the body produces less. so much so, that the heart weakens, the immune system weakens, the integrity of all the cells in the body are threaten, collagen cells lose their integrity. (The glue that binds the body together) your skin begins to sag, it is as though your body is falling apart. you look in the mirror, thinking, give me anything to put it all back together. you buy creams, ointments, all sorts of products. and you are still falling apart. every living thing on this planet needs energy, to survive. and all get it from one nutrient, (coenzyme Q 10) you can get a rich supply of coenzyme Q10. eat the hearts of other animals. the heart needs a lot of energy, so there are more concentrations of CoQ10 in the hearts of animals. In the chemical invasion epoch, we live in today. I would not eat the heart of any animal.

Today you would be eating the chemicals that cause cancer. with your rich supply of CoQ10. you would not find it in process food, as a supplement you can buy it, at a good health food store. buy a good name brand, the cheap store brands are of poor quality.

WRINKLES

Everything takes time, so if your face is falling apart. add collagen type 2 with hyaluronic acid, to your supplement list, to help repair the damage, do not sleep with your face in the pillow, putting pressure on weak skin support, will give you more wrinkles. Stay out of the sun. use a moisturizer in the summer and winter to protect from skin damage. don't wash your face with tap water use a cream.

Go to your dermatologist for acid peels. to get the spots out, use cream products with hydroquinone in it. use friendly make up, and put it on in good light, not house light. for that natural look. take cold showers, the whole body, if not then, gust the face.

Go to on line for Retin-A products use as directed to support collagen.

STOP, STUFFING YOUR MOUTH WITH GARBAGE FOOD.
None of this will work, if you keep stuffing your mouth with garbage, harmful, chemical food, you love.

VARICOSE VEINS

Buy the right support stockings, for your legs, to help varicose veins, if you have them, all of the above will help. Take grape seed extract, it has polyohenol in it that will inhibit platelet aggregation. (Blood colts) reduce inflammation, plus inhibit virus replication, interfere with cancer growth,

A high fiber diet, to prevent straining. when going to the bathroom. (that is the cause of varicose veins) when you strain, you build up enough pressure, to destroy, the valves in the veins in the legs. the pressure has to go some were, as time goes by many valves are effected, you relieve this condition by relieving constipation.

Eating less meat, and more high fiber foods, leg exercise, walk in flat shoes, or bare footed. elevate the foot of your bed a few inches. to relieve the blood pressure, while you sleep. take garlic capsules 1,000 mg per day. You do not want a blood clot, to end your life. you may say, Emilio, I begin to see clearly, the pain is gone, can you see clearly, will the pain be gone, what you stuff in your mouth, you may find hard, leaving your body, and the pressure will surely destroy all the veins, in your legs.

Did I say stuff in your mouth? I could be wrong; you may not gulp your food down. you may be the person that takes time, and chews food. the important part, of the digestion process. maybe not, in any case, take hydrochloric acid and a probiotic. like acidophilus, to add in the digestion process.

PRUITUS ANI

Do you have pruritus ani (a discharge of mucous) due to a liver problem? do you go around scratching your ass? I did, I was not a happy camper, and I ran to the supper center, to buy a liver support herbal complex. by natures bounty, plus milk thistle, and dandelion root extract, I do not have the problem today. thank GOD its part of my dark past.

THE LIVER

The human liver cleans the body of toxins, cigarette smoke, alcohol, and thousands of harmful chemicals; we are exposed to and are eating. It is an amazing organ, to complicated for any one to understand, other then its function. what we understand is the liver, overwhelmed, by harmful chemicals, is damaged. the liver is so amazing, that it can restore regenerate, most of its cells. you are probably walking around with a third of your liver working, with fat blocking circulation. if your overweight, you probably have a lot of trans fat, build up, in the liver. that will cause infection, atherosclerosis, cholesterol deposits, water build up in body tissues, all this can lead to early death.

To prevent this, stop eating refine sugar, an trans fatty acids or any arthritically produced sugar (corn syrup etc;) you can take the amino acid methionine, (to prevent fat build up in the liver) folic acid and vitamin B6, methionine, can not work with out B vitamins, to support liver health, preventing cholesterol deposits, infection, and water retention in the body. scar tissue, drug damage, from the onslaught of the chemical invasion epoch. called pathophsiology of abnormal health by traditional medicine. its a wonder your walking around at all. if the liver is impaired, then toxins build up in the body. and can cause a wide range of disease. a healthy liver is essential, to a long healthy life.

To promote the regeneration of liver cells. Take as I said a liver support herbal complex. milk thistle and dandelion root extract, garlic, and methionine, folic acid, vitamin B6.

THE MYTH OF THE BIOLOGICAL CLOCK

There is a myth in folk law in western society that old people don't need sleep, it is because old people seem to always be awake, they are about all hours of the night and day. this lends it self to the misconceptions, that a person is getting old. an old person is not active, not working, requires less energy, and there is no need for sleep. or so to speak, recharge ones batteries. another amino acid that the body produces in the brain in the pineal gland that regulates the biological clock in humans. is as time moves on, turned off. I would like to change the reference (old age) to a more positive, (as a person moves in time) the amino acid is melatonin, a deficiency, and one can wake up at different times. to reset your biological clock, and get a good nights sleep that is needed for good health. take melatonin 3mg before you go to bed. do not take melatonin in the day, or if you suffer from depression, or have an autoimmune disease. as it promotes sleep.

ARTHRITIS

Their was a time in my life. when I could not make a fist, with out pain. out in the cold, my hands would hurt. at night, I would wake up from the pain in my hands. I was thinking the beginning stages of rheumatoid arthritis. understanding the effects of this. inflammation, oproximal interphalangeal joints, swan neck deformity, the destruction of joints, fatigue due to a lot of stress. and a host of health problems.

My doctor had no idea, of what is causing all of this. to him it is all a mystery. I did not want to take dangerous pain killing drugs. I will not list the bad drugs; your doctor gives you for pain. whatever drugs he gives you. look them up on the internet; check out the side effects, it will scare the hell out of you.

At this time, I was trying to find the cause. my daughter was diagnosed with lupus. all this was giving me a lot of stress, for the stress, I would take valerian root extract. 1,500mg two or three times a day and kava before bed.

Systemic autoimmune rheumatic diseases. a mystery; is it a mystery? the immune system destroying tissue and cells. why would the immune system destroy anything? ask your doctor? I am sure your doctor would give you the answer to the mystery. he would say the immune system is protecting the body, by destroying infected cells. your doctor just solved the mystery; he should get the noble prize.

Today my daughter is in remission, and has no lupus related problems; you can buy the book lupus cure or spontaneous remission second edition, at my web site.

For my arthritis, or should I say the mystery disease. ok I am a bit apprehensive in my rhetoric, but I was in pain. for arthritis take:
Omega 3 fish oil 1,000mg per day.
Glucosamine sulfate 1,000mg per day.
Natural vitamin E d-alpha tocopherol 800mg per day.
Selenium 200mg per day.
Vitamin C 500mg per day.
Garlic 1,000mg per day.

    I would go to bed with thermo gloves on, to relieve the pain. If you have a more advance arthritis condition. go to a sports store, by a sleeping bag, put in on your bed, and sleep in it, in the morning you will be in a lot less pain.
    I stopped eating process food, junk food, frozen food, meat, dairy, and garbage food, like white bread, and all the products made with white flour, refined sugar, cold cuts, anything with artificial anything in it. I am going with what the doctor says. the immune system will destroy any cell or tissue that is infected, or invaded by garbage food, or chemicals. this could mean your whole body, is going to be destroyed, with all the garbage you eat and drink.
    Excuse me we were talking about me. In a few months, the pain was gone, in a year I was in remission, with no arthritis related problems. I kid you not my friend.

TESTOSTERONE

Every one knows about testosterone, that the body produces, as you move in time, the body produce less. this can cause many problems; one we are all concern about is prostate enlargement. this affects men over forty-five, if you have not taken saw palmetto and lycopene. see your physician; he can give you a number test. the gloved finger, blood test, ultrasound. take the entire battery of test, if you do not have a problem, or if you do, take saw palmetto and lycopene. if you have no problems, and you are down the road in time. you may want to take testosterone, replacement therapy. with saw palmetto and lycopene, there are no side effects. with (TRC) but you must be free of prostate disease.

DRUGS

Humans have been taking drugs for thousands of years. our leaders' drink alcohol in one form or another. you have had one form or another alcoholic drink, in your life. The beer in your school days.

The Romans had their wine for thousands of years. we are a young republic, founded on the consumption of alcohol. It is a mystery that the human herd animal has a need to be sedated. I can understand why you drink.

A small amount of alcohol in the body will, release a bit of adrenalin, that puts you in the fight or flight response. you feel like a big man, or woman and it increases power fancies, thoughts, frees cerebral inhibitions, not only do you feel like a big person, you think it. you are a little person, (with a need to feel powerful).understanding this, and not drinking alcohol. is the most powerful thing you can do?

To keep you alive, for a while, to give you time, to work out the power thing. take
L-glutamine 1,000 to 3.000mg capsules per day.
L-tryptophan 500mg per day.
works better with vitamin B6 100mg, and magnesium 150mg. people that drink, lose a lot of magnesium in the body.
L-cystine to prevent liver disease. taken before bed.
to repair your liver take a liver complex, milk thistle and dandelion root extract.
(all this for recovering alcoholics)
Because alcohol is a carcinogen, free radical, that causes body damage. it is essential, that you take.
Vitamin C, vitamin E, and selenium. in addition, may GOD save your soul?
You are not alone in the United States. about fifteen percent of the adult population is alcoholic. I will not talk about the kids. we even get to see our politicians, at special events, drinking, in the news, getting drunk out of their minds.

Thursday july 30 2009. The daily news a picture of president Obama with a glass of beer in his hand and the look of and alcoholic on his face

IT'S NOT OK TO DRINK ALCOHOL
Michael Daly reporting;

Quote; president Obama is expected to have a bud Light when the three sit down at a picnic table near his daughters swing set, weather permitting. un Quote

July 31, front page; daily news; president Obama, the vice president, sgt James Crowley, and Henry Louis gates jr. at a picnic table with a mugs of beers in their hands. The president and vice president Getting drunk on the job.

We have a drug addict president, who smokes and drinks, mind alteration drugs, nicotine and alcohol.
In front of his kids.

(Role model); black kids ; have a beer, get drunk, just think; you can grow up a be an alcoholic president.

alcohol even in small amounts have the effect of reducing the ability of red blood cells to carry oxygen, an adverse effect on the brains ability to make the right decisions. the X president, bush. thank GOD for the X said he was a reformed alcoholic. If we think of the state of the great republic we live in today, I would say he made a lot of bad decisions, his sole pursuit, as president. was to plunder and line the pockets of his friends in the oil an stock   business, he did a good job at the expense of great nation,

I am sure his friends will drink to that.
Most of what happens in the world is the effect of culture, disease,   famine, and a human entity with a new philosophic rhetoric.

when disease and drug affected politicians so called leaders. that are an aspect of human herd phenomenon, interfuse. the result is a cascade of catatonic events. that we all can live without, if we live at all. sure enough.

DISEASE PERVENTION

Most diseases can be prevented. a very dark area, if everyone prevented disease, the economy   of western civilization would collapse.

this book should be ban, and three hundred million people in the united states should not read this book. more likely this book will get lost in the few million that are printed every year. however, you my dear friend are reading this book. (panic liberal).

DIABETES

Doctors recommend natural medicine, dietary and lifestyle changes to cure a mystery disease. diabetes Type 2.adult-onset, non-insulin-dependent diabetes.

Diabetes type 1.juvenile diabetes cannot be cured. because the beta cells of the pancreas are destroyed. In addition, cannot produce insulin that regulates blood sugar. some children have an allergic reaction, to antigens in cow's milk. that bind with the cells of the pancreas, the immune system protecting the body destroys the infected cells of the pancreas. the child can no longer produce the hormone insulin. vital to making glucose for cells. with out life long injections, of insulin, would die in a coma.

The production of insulin is a billion dollar business, and getting bigger every year.

Breast-feeding your child is best. if not, and your child's eyes look drugged after eating a meal, aggressive behaviors, pushing the bottle away, or any behavior that's not normal. your child may have this problem. take the child to a health care professional.

Adult onset Diabetes Type 2. the major cause of diabetes type 2 is caused by the consumption of trans fatty acids and refined sugar, sugar has no nutritional value, no vitamins, is not a food, and is a chemical $C_{12}H_{22}O_{11}$. forty billion pounds of refined sugar are sold in the United States each year. it is cheap, heavy, makes money, and makes you fat. with diabetes, it is in every thing you eat. all the process food, bake food, cookies etc. are cook with vegetable oil, partially hydrogenated fats. that cause cell damage it is a major averse impact of the chemical invasion epoch. you can sell rotten food, if you put enough refined sugar in it.

Any one can go in to remission, from diabetes type 2. If it is in your mine not to suffer from, heart disease, amputation, blindness, pain, and death.

Stop eating trans fatty acids and refined sugar. Tans fats damage cell walls in the body, destroy the integrity of human cells slowly over the years, trans fats are in most of the products in your supermarket margarine is made from trans fat, its in all the process and frozen food its in all the bake goods called vegetable shortening polyunsaturated cooking oils vegetable oil corn oil partially hydrogenated vegetable oil all have trans fat the food you love.

Eat only organic raw vegetables. or organic cooked rich, carbohydrate vegetables. eat lemons to lower blood sugar but not grapefruit. eat fiber rich foods. eat brown rice, fresh fish.   no animal food. no dairy products. no process food. no salt, no refined sugar, no frozen food, no white flour, or any products made with white flour. no junk food, no white rice. no trans fats. you can eat fruits.

Your doctor cannot save you. with the little magic pills.

All your life, you have been eating many bad chemicals, in your steaks, pork chops, lamb chops, and cold cuts sandwiches. in addition, nice cold soda to wash all that garbage down. and no one told you that you are living in the chemical invasion epoch. know they will amputate your hands and feet, you will go blind, you are in pain and you will die. if you do not give up the food, you love.

Supplements every diabetic must take.

Chromium picoinate
Bilberry extract
Bitter melon juice 40ml per day, if you are not taking diabetic drugs.
Vitamin E 800mg per day.
Vitamin C 1,000mg per day.
B vitamin complex plus B 12
Vitamin B6
L-carnitine
Ginseng
Ginkgo biloba
Maitake 400mg two times a day
Quercetin
Biotin
Niacin 500mg per day.
Magnesium 300mg per day.

Their are no lessons of empowerment here, just an awareness of what you put in your mouth.

There are no lessons in stress management, just supplements to neutralize stress.

Their are no magic pills, just a will to live.

Their are no cures, just virus infected hospitals and harmful, pain killing drugs.

Their are no good laws. only lawmakers that govern and make laws under the influence of drugs.

There are no celebrations of the good life,
They celebrate the pagan ritual, New Years Eve. (Get drunk, smoke cigarettes, have sex, party all night) a collide-

oscope of culture, interfaced with chemicals, a chaotic dance of millions, to the silence, of sudden death.

It is not my purposes to cure disease. all disease can be prevented, taken in to remission, with the right diet and supplementation.

My journey is with those of you, I assume, have not yet fallen to the diseases of western civilizations. and yet. I hope that this book will reach the fifty million that will be diagnosed with heart disease, cancer, diabetes, arthritis next year.

Probably not. In any case. understanding that ageing is an abbreviation of the human herd phoneme through pathologic disease. I am force to address human disease, its cause, and how to prevent it. dealing with human systems that are interacting, and depended upon each other for good health. In addition, when something affects one system, something breaks down. and effects another system, and a disease appears. we invent a chemical to inhibit a molecule. sounds good so far?

We are definitely in the dissection room. we cannot think out of the box. things are so complex we are hopelessly confused by our failures. our success is short lived and the patient dies.

Millions are dieing every year. let us invent a new chemical, a new drug that will save humankind. yes, one is on the way, any day now, I just know it. tomorrow, tomorrow, tomorrow.

MENOPAUSE

Menopause; what is happening to me? a personality change, irregular periods, hot flashes, mood swings. As time goes by a woman stops producing eggs. the body has no need for hormones, the climacteric period. forty to seventy years of age. I am sure, woman are more eminent, then just child bearing.

Like your counterpart in the drama of herd animal phoneme, you may think, what I am about to say, is a bit abstract, even unrealistic. the body is thinking your time is up, your mission is a child bearing animal. to perpetuate the species, and all the hormones that supports that entity. Is turn off.

Your biological, genetic, clock. beckons, tomorrow is here, your time up.

At fifty years of age, you are not strong enough, to give birth to a child. the pituitary glands production of hormones and the hypothalamus, shut down. you suffer hormone deficiency. that can cause atherosclerosis, heart disease, osteoporsis, high blood pressure, obesity. It is time for you to die off.

HUMANITIES EPICENTER

I can hear the woman who epitomize woman. from, Christine De Pizan. to Simone De Beauvior, to Virginia Woolfe, to Elizabeth lady Stanton, to Susan B Anthony, to Carol Hanisch, to Sara Evans and to all at the UNs Pan Pacific South east Asia Woman's association. I need not say.

Challenge the laws written in stone. even the genetic code. everything in an exploding universe, is susceptible to change, and can be change. here we bury Hegel in a stagnant abyss, and move on.

To reduce, if not relive, the symptoms of menopause.
take;
Black Cohosh extract 250mg two or three times a day.
side effects:
no side effects at recommend doses.
Valerian root   extract 1,500mg two times a day.
side effects:
no side effects.
Kava 200mg before bed.
No side effects at recommend doses.
St johns wort 500mg per day, for depression.
Side effects:
may make the skin light sensitive.
none of this should be taken with alcohol.
eat many soy products.

Drink green tea every day, eat table mushrooms, are (anti-estrogen) most woman that eat mushrooms and drink green tea, do not get breast cancer.

If you still have problems, you should look into

hormone replacement therapy (HRT) and natural, that is true progesterone. must say micronized progesterone, or do not buy it. non-synthetic and you will have less health problems.

CANCER

your doctor may want to know if you have a history of cancer in your family. who has not, one out three people in the united States, have one form of cancer.

you have to have cancer, to be estrogen-receptor positive. tumor cells feed on estrogen to grow.

for postmenopausal and premenopausal woman. a change in diet, and supplements. will prevent breast cancer.

cancer is not a disease of genes that you inherit from some one. It's a disease that affects genes. cancer causing agents, or cancer initiators, free radicals, chemicals in food, water, air. that cause a mutation in the genetic material. (DNA) that affects the replication process. that cause malignant cells to grow.

the immune system destroys most cancer cells. traditional medicine, it's therapies weaken and damage the immune system. the only hope you have to survive.
that is why today's cancer therapy, will not cure cancer.

if the human immune system did not kill cancer cells every day, of every human's life, humans would not exist on this planet. your only hope to survive cancer, in the chemical invasion epoch you live in. is your immune system.

if you have cancer, I am talking to thirty million people. stop eating chemical garbage, become an organic vegetarian, no meat, no dairy, no refined sugar, no salt, no white flour, or any product made with white flour. no process food, no frozen food, no cold cuts, no trans fats, go to apricot seeds.com. eat many apricot seeds. take all the vitamins, herbs, nutrients, in the supplement list in this book.

You shall not be compliant and go to that medieval bacteria resistant hospital. were pieces of your body will be cut off. were you will suffer chemical burns? were you will be given narcotics? and were you will, surely die.

Surely you shall live, because you want to live, for your family, friends, for life it self. knowing your existents has an impact on every one. and every thing you interact with. and that it makes a difference.

There is no cure for cancer. understanding what the cause is and eliminating it, reinforcing your immune system, you may just go into remission.

Then and only then will you join me, young at heart. free of disease, as a man you will walk in good stride. the envy of you peers. as a woman you will radiate, a nebula of youth and beauty, to be question.

Together our hearts will be heavy. as we walk amongst the dieing, as they fall by the millions, as we reach out in vain, as they turn and will not listen, as they spit out mottos.

When it is your time to go, you go. Every one has to live, you could die in your sleep, you could be hit by a truck and die, you have to do, what you have to do. No one lives forever.

Should I waste my time and yours? and give you a list of food to eat. ok eat broccoli, its good for you. you run out buy broccoli, you eat it every day, six months later you die. the broccoli, you buy every day on sale, came from

Mexico, were they use DDT on the broccoli crops. and import it to the United States.

Not all livestock in the United States is injected with cancer causing chemicals and hormones?

Not all the six hundred thousand tons of lead. that gets into the atmosphere every day. gets into food, crops ,soil, water, and are inhaled?

Not all the one hundred and thirty four million tons of refined sugar are consumed buy Americans?

Not all of the ten billion pounds of pesticide, herbicides, and fungicide, produced every year are used on crops in the united states. just two billion pounds are used in the united states. three point seven million pounds are used every year on tomatoes alone. seven hundred pounds per acre on potato's.

The amount of harmful chemicals, misguided humans consume today. Is a staggering apocalypse of disease pain and death.

In a million years of human evolution. we have today, a genetically programmed macro parasite. born with a inclination; to love or hate, to be predator or pray, to plan the annihilation of a nation, or the preservation of a nation.

In the chemical invasion epoch we live in. humans have chosen extermination. an awareness, of the pathological impact of the chemicals, we consume. and a sociological impact, of that awareness, on the genetically programmed, human macro parasite. that is adaptable, capable of change. over long periods of time. can we change. can we adapt. do we have the time? technology is moving at lighting speed.

Thousands if not millions of tons of new harmful

chemicals are consume each year. humans are considered lest of an entity. and more of a consumer of product.

Humans are an entity, a miracle of interacting events. the destruction of planet earth, is witness to those events.

How can you and I, even think we can live a long life in the chemical invasion epoch we live in.

When sodium nitrate is ingested, it is converted in to substances called nitrosamines. that are carcinogenic and cause stomach cancer, and all the rheumatic diseases. rheumatoid arthritis, osteoarthritis, juvenile arthritis, systemic lupus, gout, ankylosis sodalities, fibrositis, psoriatic arthritis.

A cold cut hero sandwich, ham and cheese, letters and tomatoes. on a half a loaf of Italian bread. a bottle of beer, or a soda. the good food I love to eat. with out sodium nitrate, their would be no nice fresh cold cuts; to eat.

Doctors dismiss the idea that the cause of rheumatic disease is carcinogens. because their pay check comes from the same people, that produce product and drugs that are carcinogenetic. they rationalize to protect their sanity. and say rheumatic diseases are mysterious diseases.

The most dangerous, and really stupid thing to do, is to try to suppress the immune system.

There are ten trillion immune cells, a hundred million different B cells, coursing around in blood and lymphatic system. and that's just B cells.

The adrenal corticosteroids, used in traditional medicine today. prednisone, cortisone, fludrocortisones, etc. do not work. the patients condition degenerates. the patients dies. from a mysterious diseases. that we don't want to talk about, because it hurts our brain, and our paycheck, to admit the truth.

This can make a person mad with anger, at doctors. . and yet. It is the anger in a person that can heal disease. the mental disposition, of a person. the biochemical, reaction of anger. that sets one on a path to remission.

Get mad, get angry, demand the truth. stop eating the food they make taste good. that gives you pains in your hands, pains in your back, pains in your stomach, pains in your chest, pains in your heart, and pains in your ass. prednisone cures nothing.

Get mad, it is your right to know the truth. the cause of disease in your hands, the cause of disease in your back, the cause of disease in your stomach, the cause of disease in your chest, and the cause of heart disease.

Tell me prednisone will cure me. if not, then stick the prednisone up "your; give me not chemical pain and death. give me a cure, or give me the door.

I have the right to be mad, angry, piss off at the bullshit you doctors don't want to talk about. I need real help and I need it now; today. is their any part of that you do not understand.

I feel better; yes. "yes; I feel better. I will not eat the chemical garbage. you call cold cuts, you call natural frozen food, you call natural process food, you call natural canned food, you call food.

It has to many chemicals in it and you know it. it is all part of the chemical invasion epoch we live in. created by the food and drug industries to make money and money they make, lots of it. for they are true macro parasites, indeed. they make millions of dollars, from the millions of people that eat chemicals. and millions of people get diseases, from eating chemicals. they make millions, selling drugs to people that get diseases from chemicals. and millions of people die. they are   true macro parasites indeed. and yet;

    We are all macro parasites. the good part of this story is we live in a great democracy you can eat or not eat. no one can force you to do anything. I will say to you that you will live longer and healthier if you were a vegetarian but that is up to you.

MOLECULES OF DEATH

Every one has at one time or another, listen to someone talk about mad cow.

What is mad cow. a neurodegenerative disease Transmissible spongiform encephalopathies (TSEs)

Today one may say he or she died from Creutzfeldt-jakob disease (CJD)

The scary part, of all of this is that something adverse that affects molecular structures in humans. has appeared and the effects of it is that it dissolves the neuron structures in human brains. called the prion disease.

Dr Stanley B Prusiner. won the Nobel prize in physiology or medicine. In 1997 for his research.

My hero was Daniel Carleton Gajdusek won the Nobel prize in physiology or medicine in 1976 for his research for the disease kuru

In New Guinea. People practice cannibalism is was the first prion disease. They would eat the brains of people that were infected with a disease called kuru, and they would get the disease

Daniel Carleton Gajdusek suggested that if a cow had the disease, and the cow was grounded up and fed to another cow, or a dairy cow, that cow would get infected. and in turn humans eat the cow or drink cows milk would get the disease.

Thus assuming rendered animals used as feed for cows, chickens, an all live stock.

in the united states. today millions of tons of dead animals, chickens, cows, dogs and cats from shelters. From slaughterhouses blood, entrails, byproducts from the food processing industries. and wastes products like sludge or maggot infested dead diseased animals, rodents. billions of pounds of grease and tallow.

are process as feed. proteins, for live stock and dairy cattle. all this good stuff is process in the disposal operations of the rendering industry, today, as I speak; are made into feed formulations for chickens and cows. that we eat. and cows milk that you drink.

Assuming one dead animal has bovine spongiform encephalopathy.(BSE) and is process into feed. gets into the human food supply. human brains will dissolve.

It is a time bomb, that is happening or is it happening? Their was one case reported in the united states.

In 1996 Oprah Winfrey talked about cattle being fed to cattle. she was sued. she will not talk about it again. shut your mouth girl.

There is strong evidence that these manifestations are a direct result of cannibalism. to us the evidence is just manifestations.

Thousand of cases of bovine spongiform encephalopathy (BSE)   better known as mad cow disease or creutzfeldt-jakob disease (CJD) has been reported in the united kingdom and more to come because of the long incubation period of the disease.

May be caused by the consumption of BSE contaminated meat and bone supplements in cattle feed. the united states and Canada ban feeding of ruminant products cattle, sheep, and goats, to ruminant live stock cattle sheep and goats etc. of cause there is no real way to enforce a ban. if there is a real ban. no way to prove, or any way to detect dead disease ruminant animals, that are in protein finished feed. billions of dollars at risk, is any one paying attention, don't worry theirs no real proof of transmissible mad cow disease or any of the prion diseases (CJD) etc. with the long incubation period of the disease, you probably die of heart disease, before the disease takes affect.

With all the chemical garbage you put in your mouth. what difference would it make.

go have your barbeque, steaks, chickens, and don't forget the franks and soda. enjoy your life, you never know, your brain may dissolve just like that. It may be psychosomatic, maybe you just inherited it from your family, maybe its sorcery, ask your doctor I'm sure he will come up with something like, its in the family, or it's a mystery.

If you want my opinion, I would say it's a alien plot to destroy the world as we know it.

GOUT

Gout: to much uric acid, or your body can not get rid of uric acid and it builds up. gout can go in to remission with a change in diet. stop eating high protein fat foods,

Stop eating meat animal or dairy products stop drinking alcohol, eat a lot of organic celery, cherries, tomatoes, cherry juice, raw carrots, brown rice, vegetable juice, to neutralize the uric acid. Take all the supplements in this book for anti ageing. don't eat refined sugar, salt, or any food that you love. to get rid of kidney stones take vitamin B 6 and magnesium hydroxide every day it works better then the thiazides drugs that your doctor gives you that promotes gout. raises uric acid levels in the body.

COMPASSION

It is with compassion that I contemplate disease produced in a sick society that consume alcohol drugs and chemicals.

It is with compassion that I contemplate sick politicians and celebrities that consume alcohol drugs and chemicals.

It is with compassion that I contemplate sick liberal news papers saying its ok and fun that our leaders and celebrities consume alcohol drugs and chemicals.

It is with compassion that I contemplate a healthy person saying it is not ok, to consume alcohol drugs and chemicals period.

DISEASE PREVENTION

This is the part of the book that makes it all happen. as a man you will walk in good stride the envy of your peers.
as a woman you will radiate a nebula of youth and beauty to be question.

the first understand that needs to be made clear is that vitamins, nutrients, herbs and minerals. are find by themselves. together they interact support and enhance each others effects. it is when you take them in combinations, that the you get the best benefit from them.

Should be taken after dinner, unless you can take them throughout the day, if not after dinner is best.

Take natural vitamins, not synthetic. for the added benefits of natures substances as bioflavonoid in natural vitamin C from rose hips. and tocopherols in natural vitamin E, etc.

I talked about human cell integrity, that is compromised by trans fatty acids, free radicals, harmful chemicals, that get into the layers of cells disrupt if not destroy the cells.

The driving force of all healthy cells in the human body is its energy component. that is a nutrient; Coenzyme Q 10, (CoQ10). no one could survive with out it, and when it is depleted in the body, all disease states appear. the lack of CoQ10 in the body, and the impact of trans fatty acids, free radicals, and harmful chemicals.

And heart cells, immune system cells, all major organ cells. are affected, the integrity and proper function of each cell is threaten. leading to disease and early death.

the body produces CoQ10, as humans move in time the body turns off the process that produces CoQ10 in the body. all major organs are weaken by the lack of CoQ10 in the body, and are susceptible to disease.

To prevent this if not slow this human phoneme of spiraling disease, pain an eventual death.

A combination of
CoQ10-90mg per day
Natural vitamin E- 800mg per day
Selenium 200mg per day
Vitamin C 500mg per day

Working together, CoQ10, vitamin E, selenium, and vitamin C. will neutralize free radicals and harmful chemicals, restore energy to every cell.

Trans fatty acids, my friend, you must read the labels, if it says no trans fatty acids; its false advertising. Today the USDA says it is legal to say no trans fatty acids in big letters. if your product says, in little small barely reader able; at the bottom of the package, up to 0.5 grams of TFAs.

It still has trans fatty acids that are not real fats and get into cells, create problems. and in time destroy cells, you may die if enough of your heart cells are destroyed.

Come on, most of all the company's that cook food. process food, frozen food, chips, cookies, baked products, etc. use cheap, partially hydrogenated vegetable oils.

Well not all; their are some company's that do not use cheap trans fatty acid oils, to cook their food. of cause, up to 0.5grams of TFAs would not be on their labels.

Check the whole package, they like to hide, the words up to 0.5grams of TFAs.

Did you ever read a label, that said potato chips cooked in olive oil. that is the only chips I will eat, or I will not eat them at all, period.

Hey I don't want to get a heart attack, from trans fatty acids. that are used to cook all the box food in your supermarket. even the nice hot cooked food that you can buy at the supermarket, so you don't have to cook dinner, they use cheap mazola vegetable oil, I   asked, I even went behind the counter and looked, yes.

If you stop eating TFAs, in time your whole body will feel better, as the bad fat leaves the body. and the body repairs it self. Hopefully; if its not to late? your reading this book, your still alive, in pain, but still alive, there is hope.

All the systemic autoimmune rheumatic diseases are described as mysterious diseases by your doctor.

He is not going to tell you that your immune system is attacking all the pollution that gets in you body from tap water that you brush your teeth with, to the air you breath, the dirt and chemicals in the process food you eat, refined sugar, and chemical imitation sugar that is in all the food you eat.

He's not going to tell you, the cold cuts have dangerous chemical preservatives. he's not going to tell you, the problem is what you put in your mouth.

Because he has no clue? how dangerous chemicals in food affect the human body is not in the medical books he studied to become a doctor. he may take a short class on nutrition. that may be about cholesterol. that's it.

It is a mystery to me; with the new peptide chemistry science, and it's

scientific proof that there are receptors on every cell in the human body, affected by wide range of neuro-peptides chemicals hormones insulin etc.

scientific proof that the body is regulated by a flow of information, in the form of body chemistry, to every cell in the human body.

It is a mystery to me that traditional medicine has not giving way to the neuropsychopharmacologists that offer

scientific proof that every human cell has receptors. that all human cells communicate with each other

scientific proof that the immune system will produce chemicals in the form of neuro-peptides that will send out information.

Scientific proof that this chemical information will determine the health or the destruction of every cells.

I know this new science will prevail because it has all the answers to all the diseases.

And if you are a little hungry research scientist that can win the noble prize in this challenging science of cell, peptides, receptors, molecules,

Understanding that this new science of cell chemical information processing and the scientific proof that it exist. takes on a wide range of information processing involving all of the human senses and converting it into chemical data in a language that only at this time the body understands and reacts to. this chemical language can be understood with the help of today's computer technology.

I shall leave that to the little hungry research scientist; that noble prize winner of tomorrow.

It is no mystery to me that this new science, will in time replace traditional medicine.

In that day their will be no need for bacteria and virus infected hospitals. that humans are dissected, drugged, cut, burned, and;

the only reaction to the body, is that the sensitive system of cells and it's information processing chemicals are damage, disrupted, destroyed, the body dies.

The dark age of traditional medicine is at it's END.
For, I have spoken

Let us deal with today's pain, and not tomorrows, medical science.

Do you want to live with out pain?

Do you want to live with out disease?

Do you want to live with out depression?

Do you want to live with out the food you love?

Do you want to live to see your children's children grow?

Do you want to see a bird fly, a leaf fall, a sun set, a sun rise, a winter storm, a summer breeze, a butterfly, alight on a leaf.

Do you want to live?

You can say something really stupid. at this point in time, like. every one has to go sometime, the.

If your not really stupid that is you don't say stupid things like, you can get hit with a truck and die in a minute.

To all the people that are not really stupid.

To all the people that are not really stupid, that read food labels.

To all the people that are not really stupid, that put things in their mouth that taste good, and makes them fat.

To all the people that are not really stupid, that think their doctor can cure them.

To all the people that are not really stupid, that eat food loaded with salt and refined sugar. because they are addicted to it.

To all the people that are not really stupid, that drink coffee because they are addicted to it.

To all the people that are not really stupid, that are caught in the chemical invasion epoch and don't understand it.

To all the people that are not really stupid, that want to change, and want to live in good health.

To all the people that are not really stupid,

STAND UP AND JOIN ME TODAY, TAKE CHARGE.

Eat lots of food, yes, the right food.

Take lots of nutrients', vitamins, supplements, the right, nutrients, vitamins, and supplements.

Every receptor on every cell in your body is waiting, for.

the right combinations of the right food.

the right combinations of vitamins.

The right combinations nutrients.

The right combinations of supplements

Every receptor on every cell in waiting for life giving energy, life supporting body chemicals. that can be processed for the good of the body's health. for human survival, humans have a neurochemistry that is to complex for today's medical science to want to understand. the effects of neuropeptides and neurophysiological changes that determine every aspect of human health and behavior. and the recent scientific proof of cell receptors and neurochemical reactions in all parts of the body in an amazing system of interacting processing information technology on a biochemical level.

Lift up your ears, open your eyes, doctors. stop giving drugs to patients, in watch and wait therapy.

It is like adding a virus to a highly sophisticated computer system.

Lift up your ears, and open your eyes surgeons, stop cutting, burning and adding gadgets to patients.

It is like taking parts out, interrupting, damaging systems and adding gadgets to a highly sophisticated computer system, that you know very little about.

we all know, what happens to the patients.

we all know, what happens to the sophisticated human system.

we all want to know why, more then fifty million patients, die of heart disease, every year?

In the united states.

EXERCISE

Ok everybody go out and ride in that bicycle path by the highway or run in the path by the highway or walk in the path by the highway. anyone can tell I am from New York city, in New York city every one gets their exercise by a highway or alongside cars in traffic, is it because they are all nuts, out of their mines, they are running alongside cars in traffic, is any one thinking, carbon monoxide

poison. It's a good idea to exercise, but please; not in traffic.
a better idea is the Taoist tai chi society of the USA.
Tai chi for health. or any good health exercise, class.
that you can get into every week.

UNDERSTANDING PAIN

I would like to summarize what has been said in this book, then give you all the combinations of supplements, to take every day, beginning with a clear understanding of pain.

Human pain is the body's, alarm system. telling the person that something is wrong. well, we all know that. this we can call body intellect. if you damage your toe, the body sends a message to your conscience mind telling you. you need to do something about your toe. if there is a break in the skin the body's intellect will alert the immune system. the immune system will react, to protect the body. from harmful bacteria. well, we all know that.

How this happens is astonishing; it happens in an instant. the biochemical information processing technology is amazing so amazing it is dismissed. a human cell is damaged in your toe and in a instant you feel a lot of pain.

If you spill hot water on your hand, you will know about it, in an instant. you will feel the pain.

Well, we all know this. that amazing instant, that human biochemical, astonishing information processing technology. the pain you feel, can not be dismissed.

This amazing body intellect that is part of every cell in the human body will in an instant, let you know a cell is damage. that astonishing information processing body intellect will let you know, in pain. That cells are damaged.

In essence a damage human cell is the catalyst that will provoke a pain response in the body.

The entire body is receptor sensitive, when you touch something you know it, you are conscious of it in an instant. if the integrity of a healthy cell is threaten, or damaged. any cell in the entire body; all are receptor sensitive. and will provoke a pain response.

Humans are a, sophisticated interactive invormental organism. that will react to any chemical it comes in contact with. that reaction can be pain or repair, death or life, receptors on every cell will process incoming chemical information, will dictate a chemical response.

Left to its own amazing biochemical technologies. can reject, neutralize, stabilizes, alert the immune system to attack, incoming harmful chemicals.

The onslaught of harmful drugs, shocking surgery, and gadgets. implemented by the so called modern medical science of today, disrupt, inhibited, undermine, and destroy, the natural process of the body to protect it self. The result is out of control disease and eminent death.

Pain is the reaction of the body intellect, provoked by a harmful impact of internal or external stimuli, to receptor conscience cells. that in response, create neuropetides. (chemical Information to the immune system) that will determine the life or death of the cells.

The immune system is programmed to protect healthy cells in the entire body,

The immune system is programmed to destroy cells that are not healthy in the entire body if the integrity of a cell is challenge by harmful chemicals in the food you eat or air you breath.

"Come on; all of this is so simple to understand a child could understand this,

Seventy five million people a year get heart attacks.

Fifty million people a year are diagnose with cancer.

Twenty five million people a year are diagnose with diabetes.

One hundred fifty million people in the united states are in pain.

More then two hundred million people in the united states are over weight.

Millions of people die from disease every year in the united states. more then all the wars ever.

What are we talking about, human cells with receptors, chemical information communicators, Synapses, ganglia, neuropeptides, axons, dendrites, molecules. Processing memory.

How do you think you are able to walk, talk, smell, touch, taste, have sight, think.

Do you think this amazing supper high technological system that operates on a chemical base using electrical impulses, an unimaginable computer chemical driven system.

Do you think that this system would not detect a harmful chemical that is in the food you have eating. that has invaded cells in the tissues of your arthritis hands, knees, arms, back, an not send a message to the immune system to destroy the tissues, think again. The proof of this, is the pain you feel.

What part of all of this, do you not, understand?

FOOD

I will not tell you what not to eat, that's crazy, who am I to tell you what to eat, or not to eat.

I will tell you, what I eat and what I will not eat.

I will not eat beef that is injected with harmful chemicals

I will not eat pork that is injected with harmful water and chemicals, and its not even spring water.

I will not eat boneless chicken breast that is injected with harmful water an chemicals, and its not even spring water.

I will not eat any live stock that is raised on process feed.

I will not eat process food that is made with harmful chemicals, loaded with refined sugar, salt, cooked in cheap trans fat oil, water, and its not even spring water.

I will not eat frozen process food that is made with harmful chemicals cooked in cheap trans fat oil, loaded with refined sugar, salt, water, and its not even spring water.

I will not drink dirty chemical treated tap water.

I will not eat any product that in made whit white, so called enrich flour, with harmful chemicals added.

I will not eat any product with refined sugar or sugars made from corn syrup etc,

I will not eat any product loaded with salt. Cooked in cheap trans fat vegetable oil, like potato chips.

I will not eat any product that has sodium nitrate in it like cold cuts, or franks, hams, etc. that cause cancer.

I will not eat any caned product with chemicals, loaded with refined sugar, salt, water, and its not even spring water.

I will not eat in a dirty restaurant or coffee shop

I will not eat any of this because I do not want to get a heart attack, cancer, diabetes, arthritis, gout, etc.

I will not eat any of it because the body intellect,(the receptor sensitive cells in the whole body); will process information to the immune system to attack every cell that is effected by all of this so called food that I will not eat.

To maintain the integrity and health of all the cells in my body.

I will read every label of every food product that I consume

I will cook all my food in olive oil.

I will eat lots of raw USA organic fruits and vegetables. that I like.

I will drink USA organic juices.

I will drink USA organic milk.

I will eat USA organic potatoes, brown rice, cooked in spring water.

I will cook fresh fish in olive oil.

I will eat USA organic peanut butter. On organic whole wheat bread, more protein then a steak.

I will eat USA organic cereal.

I will eat USA organic peanut butter.

I will eat the thousands of USA organic products that I like.

I understand I live in a dangerous place, this planet earth.

There are chemical poisons, in the air.

There are chemical poisons, in the food.

There are chemical poisons produced in my body, reactions, to people and events.

There are chemical poisons in the drugs the doctor gives people.

THE OPTIMIST

I understand I can change this place, into a healthy place for me. not for anyone, for my self, I do it every day.

I am not going to tell every one to stop driving their car. that's crazy. I drive a car.

I am not going to tell every one to stop putting chemicals in food. that's crazy.

I am not going to tell doctors to take the chemical poisons out of the drugs he gives people, that crazy.

I am not going to tell people to stop smoking, that's crazy.

I am not going to tell people to stop drinking beer, that's crazy.

It's a crazy world we live in, and crazy people do crazy things, and get crazy pain and die crazy fast.

(that's their problem)

NEUTRALIZE POISON CHEMICALS

If you live in a big city. I do not have to explain air pollution, from cars, trucks, factories, etc.

carbon monoxide poisoning will reduce the capacity of red blood cells to deliver oxygen to the body tissues. by binding to cell receptors that normally bind to oxygen in the whole body. the heart, lungs, brain etc.

Treatment, one would have to breath in a lot of pure oxygen to maintain the integrity of affected cells and to compete for oxygen binding receptors that carbon monoxide may bind to, of cause not breathing in carbon monoxide. Carbon monoxide depletes vitamin C in the body. you need to take a lot of natural vitamin C capsules or drink a lot of organic USA orange juice with that pure oxygen.

I am sure that all the doctors will agree to what has been said about carbon monoxide poisoning.

There are hundreds of thousands of harmful chemicals that we consume every day in the chemical invasion epoch.

There are harmful chemicals you eat, breath, smell, Touch, that bind with receptors in the tissues in your body that are the cause of your arthritis, cancer, diabetes, heart disease, lupus, gout. etc.

One has only to eliminate the harmful chemicals that has, bonded to the receptors of the cells, repair the damage, and pain will stop and the disease will go in to remission.

or, prevent the harmful chemical from binding to receptor on cells. In our primitive state of human biotechnology we need not understand how garlic works better as a cure for tuberculosis then most treatments. that it works as a antibiotic. that it works is the reality we must live with. It is not what your doctor has to say about non prescription drugs or food that will save your life. It is what works that saves your life. eating a lot of organic clean fresh garlic works, not the cheap on sale garlic that has thousands of added chemicals, pesticides, that only the boys at the FDA know about, hey the farm boys have to keep pest out of the crops. millions of tons of fresh chemical sprayed fruit and vegetables that you can buy on sale, half price, buy one get one free.

If you don't like garlic in your food then buy garlic extract capsules 1,000 mg per day.

I use organic garlic in my food, and I take garlic extract capsules.

It is difficult if not imposable to neutralize the harmful effects of a person that consumes fifty pounds of pesticides, seventy five pounds of refined sugar, sixty pounds of salt, a hundred pounds of food additives, forty pounds of food color, carbon monoxide, and more chemical poisons a year.

I can imagine, you want to live a long life.

I can imagine, you want to lose weight.

I can imagine, you want to feel good about the way you look.

I can imagine, you want to be free of disease.

I can imagine, you will learn to eat the food your body needs and not the food that taste good, that you like to eat, that is killing you.

I can imagine, you in a good healthy body, looking

twenty years younger then you are.

Can you imagine, the way I feel.

If you can imagine it, you can live it.

Some really important foods to eat every day are raw organic fruits and vegetables take your pick all have special benefit's the more the better. the vegetable fiber alone will raise the good HDL in your body every one knows the health benefit of that.

Add organic onions and peppers to your cooked foods always cook in olive oil for special health benefits. Onions like garlic work as   anticoagulants peppers have special benefits especially if they are hot peppers.

It's fun when you can eat all the good foods and not gain weight,

It's fun when you can eat a lot of good food every day and not gain weight.

It's fun to see your self lose weight look good for the first time in your life.

It's fun when every one wants to look as good as you.

It's funny, I have not eaten refined sugar, or salt, in my food, for such a long time. that I can detect even small amounts in any food I eat.

In the morning I eat big bowl of organic cereal I add organic raisins, fruit, organic no fat milk, I drink 8oz bottle of spring water. I toast, a product called yoga bread, by a company called, the baker, it has lot of good plant seeds in it, sesame, poppy, pumpkin, flaxseed, whole wheat with some organic butter.

The most important aspect of human health, can cure all the inflections of disease, balance human chemistry, prevent disease, promote health, slow the aging process, is consuming plant life. the most successful prescription drugs are made from plants, all the pain killers are made from plants. you can change your life from unhealthy to radiant health from tired to vitality it's all in the plants.

And exotic plants are disappearing, from plant earth fast, when all the exotic plant life disappears, humans will become extinct.

Because the cure in plant life, they will need to fine, to cure, the new plague, will have if not today, become extinct.

THE PERPETUATION OF HEALTY BODY PARTS BY CONSUMING PLANTS

L-lysine: 500mg per day.
L-Arginine: 750mgt L-Citrulline 250mgt complex.
Lecithin choline: 1200mg per day.
Milk thistle: 175mg per day.
Green tea extract: 300mg per day.
Folic acid: 400 mg per day.
Vitamin C: 500mg per day.
Garlic: capsules 1,000mg per day.
Biberry extract: 125 mg per day astragals 1,500 mg per day.
Astragals: 1,500 mg per day.
Grape sees extract: 150mg per day.
Omega 3 fish oil: 1,000 mg per day.
Flaxseed oil: 1,000 per day.
A complex of glucosamine chondroitin vitamin C hyaluronic acid and more that will address arthritis, a product called,(osteo bi-flex joint shield formula).
A complex of calcium magnesium zinc with vitamin D by natures bounty.
Vitamin B6:   100mg per day.
Lutein: 5 to 20 mg per day.
CoQ10:   90mg per day.
Selenium: 200mg per day.
Natural vitamin E; d-alpha tocopherol: 800mg per day.
Collagen 2 with hyaluronic acid
Cretine: 3to5 grams. Per day.
Ginkgo biloba as a tea two or three times a day or an extract 60mg per day.

Gotu kola as a tea two or three times a day or extract 60mg per day.
Kava as a tea or extract 140mg per day, taken before bed .
(There are no side effects, to all supplements as recommended.)

    Eat raw organic carrots, broccoli, lettuce, baby spinach, onions, celery.
lots of natural beta carotene. Corn on the cob
Brown rice.

    there are hundreds of organic new products I live in New York city, I buy most of my organic foods at a giant supermarket called, Shop Rite. they have a large variety of organic fruits, vegetables, and organic   box foods, cereals etc.

    Fresh fish, more then just food, fresh fish is a natural pharmaceutical that will prevent and cure all disease as it's natural omega 3 oil and other chemical sustenances not yet discovered, infuse in to all cells in the body, vital to long healthy life.

    You work for your money why spend it on food color, chemicals, sugar, salt. white bread, soda, potato chips, etc. that in time will kill you. If you don't change the food you eat, you will not reach sixty years old with out a disease. If you get to seventy it will be in pain every day.

READ THE FOOD LABLES
THE LIFE YOU SAVE, MAY BE?

A, CHILD.
A, WIFE.
A, HUSBAN.
A, SON.
A, DAUGTHER .
A, MOTHER.
A, FATHER.
A, FRIEND.
If you don't read the food labels all will pass, non will last.

      The time has come to talk of many things.
A liberation of your fixed, conforming, immature, existence. Toward a healthy mature development, in that stage.
      As a man you will walk in a stride to the envy of your peers.
      As a woman you will radiated a nebula of youth and beauty to be question?

   May GOD an your body intellect, grant you good health and long life.

Emilio Garcia

www.ingramcontent.com/pod-product-compliance
Lightning Source LLC
Chambersburg PA
CBHW081213180526
45170CB00006B/2321